The Ultimate Diabetic Cooking Bo

Tasty and Affordable Diabetic Recipe:
the Right Foot

Millie Lawrence

Table of contents

WHOLE-GRAIN PANCAKES 9

BUCKWHEAT GROUTS BREAKFAST BOWL 12

PEACH MUESLI BAKE 14

STEEL-CUT OATMEAL BOWL WITH FRUIT AND NUTS 17

WHOLE-GRAIN DUTCH BABY PANCAKE... 19

MUSHROOM, ZUCCHINI, AND ONION FRITTATA............................ 22

SPINACH AND CHEESE QUICHE 25

SPICY JALAPENO POPPER DEVILED EGGS 28

LOVELY PORRIDGE 30

SALTY MACADAMIA CHOCOLATE SMOOTHIE 32

BASIL AND TOMATO BAKED EGGS 34

CINNAMON AND COCONUT PORRIDGE 36

AN OMELET OF SWISS CHARD.. 38

CHEESY LOW-CARB OMELET 40

YOGURT AND KALE SMOOTHIE.. 42

BACON AND CHICKEN GARLIC WRAP 44

GRILLED CHICKEN PLATTER 46

PARSLEY CHICKEN BREAST 48

MUSTARD CHICKEN 50

BALSAMIC CHICKEN 52

GREEK CHICKEN BREAST 55

CHIPOTLE LETTUCE CHICKEN... 57

STYLISH CHICKEN-BACON WRAP.. 60

HEALTHY COTTAGE CHEESE PANCAKES.. 62

AVOCADO LEMON TOAST 64

HEALTHY BAKED EGGS... 66

QUICK LOW-CARB OATMEAL 69

TOFU AND VEGETABLE SCRAMBLE 71

BREAKFAST SMOOTHIE BOWL WITH FRESH BERRIES 74

CHIA AND COCONUT PUDDING 76

TOMATO AND ZUCCHINI SAUTÉ 78

STEAMED KALE WITH MEDITERRANEAN DRESSING 80

HEALTHY CARROT MUFFINS 82

VEGETABLE NOODLES STIR-FRY 85

CAULIFLOWER MAC & CHEESE 88

EASY EGG SALAD 91

BAKED CHICKEN LEGS 93

CREAMED SPINACH 95

STUFFED MUSHROOMS 97

BERRY-OAT BREAKFAST BARS 99

WHOLE-GRAIN BREAKFAST COOKIES 102

PEANUT BUTTER BARS 105

ZUCCHINI BREAD PANCAKES 107

Blueberry Breakfast Cake

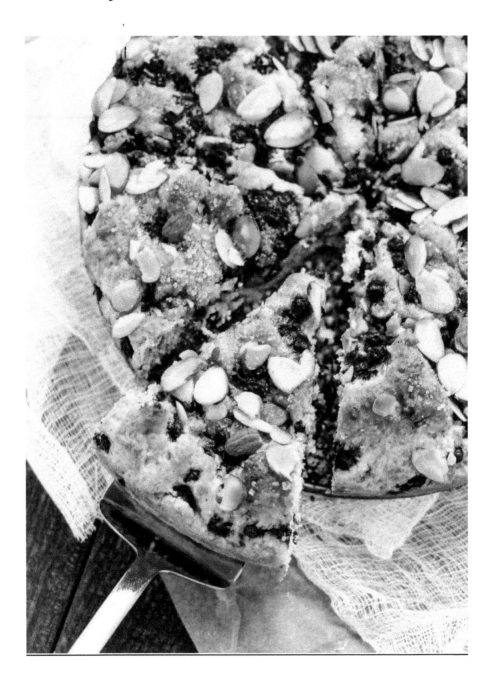

Preparation Time : 15 minutes

Cooking Time : 45 minutes

Servings : 12

Ingredients :

For the topping

- ¼ cup finely chopped walnuts
- 1/2 teaspoon ground cinnamon
- 2 tablespoons butter, chopped into small pieces
- 2 tablespoons sugar

For the cake

- Nonstick cooking spray
- 1 cup whole-wheat pastry flour
- 1 cup oat flour
- ¼ cup sugar
- 2 teaspoons baking powder
- 1 large egg, beaten
- 1/2 cup skim milk
- 2 tablespoons butter, melted
- 1 teaspoon grated lemon peel
- 2 cups fresh or frozen blueberries

Directions:

To make the topping

1. In a small bowl, stir together the walnuts, cinnamon, butter, and sugar. Set aside.

To make the cake

1. Preheat the oven to 350f. Spray a 9-inch square pan with cooking spray. Set aside.

2. In a large bowl, stir together the pastry flour, oat flour, sugar, and baking powder.

3. Add the egg, milk, butter, and lemon peel, and stir until there are no dry spots.

4. Stir in the blueberries, and gently mix until incorporated. Press the batter into the prepared pan, using a spoon to flatten it into the dish.

5. Sprinkle the topping over the cake.

6. Bake for 40 to 45 minutes, until a toothpick inserted into the cake comes out clean, and serve.

Nutrition : Calories: 177; Total Fat: 7g; Saturated Fat: 3g; Protein: 4g; Carbs: 26g; Sugar: 9g; Fiber: 3g; Cholesterol: 26mg; Sodium: 39mg

Whole-Grain Pancakes

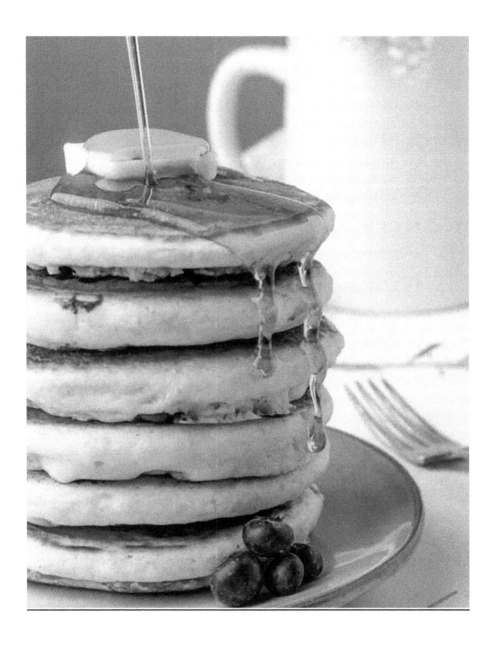

Preparation Time : 10 minutes

Cooking Time : 15 minutes

Servings : 4 to 6

Ingredients:

- 2 cups whole-wheat pastry flour
- 4 teaspoons baking powder
- 2 teaspoons ground cinnamon
- 1/2 teaspoon salt
- 2 cups skim milk, plus more as needed
- 2 large eggs
- 1 tablespoon honey
- Nonstick cooking spray
- Maple syrup, for serving
- Fresh fruit, for serving

Directions:

1. In a large bowl, stir together the flour, baking powder, cinnamon, and salt.

2. Add the milk, eggs, and honey, and stir well to combine. If needed, add more milk, 1 tablespoon at a time, until there are no dry spots and you have a pourable batter.

3. Heat a large skillet over medium-high heat, and spray it with cooking spray.

4. Using a ¼-cup measuring cup, scoop 2 or 3 pancakes into the skillet at a time. Cook for a couple of minutes, until bubbles form on the surface of the pancakes, flip, and cook for 1 to 2 minutes more, until golden brown and cooked through. Repeat with the remaining batter.

5. Serve topped with maple syrup or fresh fruit.

Nutrition : Calories: 392; Total Fat: 4g; Saturated Fat: 1g; Protein: 15g; Carbs: 71g; Sugar: 11g; Fiber: 9g; Cholesterol: 95mg; Sodium: 396mg

Buckwheat Grouts Breakfast Bowl

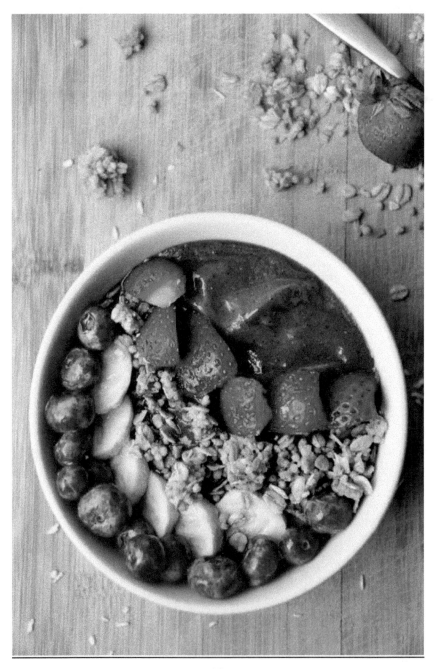

Preparation Time : 5 minutes, plus overnight to soak

Cooking Time : 10 to 12 minutes

Servings : 4

Ingredients:

- 3 cups skim milk
- 1 cup buckwheat grouts
- ¼ cup chia seeds
- 2 teaspoons vanilla extract
- 1/2 teaspoon ground cinnamon
- Pinch salt
- 1 cup water
- 1/2 cup unsalted pistachios
- 2 cups sliced fresh strawberries
- ¼ cup cacao nibs (optional)

Directions :

1. In a large bowl, stir together the milk, groats, chia seeds, vanilla, cinnamon, and salt. Cover and refrigerate overnight.

2. The next morning, transfer the soaked mixture to a medium pot and add the water. Bring to a boil over medium-high heat, reduce the heat to maintain a simmer, and cook for 10 to 12 minutes, until the buckwheat is tender and thickened.

3. Transfer to bowls and serve, topped with the pistachios, strawberries, and cacao nibs (if using).

Nutrition : Calories: 340; Total Fat: 8g; Saturated Fat: 1g; Protein: 15g; Carbs: 52g; Sugar: 14g; Fiber: 10g; Cholesterol: 4mg; Sodium: 140mg

Peach Muesli Bake

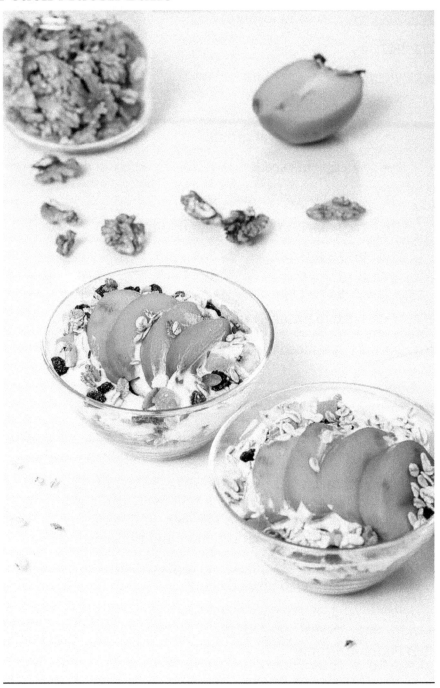

Preparation Time : 10 minutes

Cooking Time : 40 minutes

Servings : 8

Ingredients :

- Nonstick cooking spray
- 2 cups skim milk
- 11/2 cups rolled oats
- 1/2 cup chopped walnuts
- 1 large egg
- 2 tablespoons maple syrup
- 1 teaspoon ground cinnamon
- 1 teaspoon baking powder
- 1/2 teaspoon salt
- 2 to 3 peaches, sliced

Directions :

1. Preheat the oven to 375f. Spray a 9-inch square baking dish with cooking spray. Set aside.

2. In a large bowl, stir together the milk, oats, walnuts, egg, maple syrup, cinnamon, baking powder, and salt. Spread half the mixture in the prepared baking dish.

3. Place half the peaches in a single layer across the oat mixture.

4. Spread the remaining oat mixture over the top. Add the remaining peaches in a thin layer over the oats. Bake for 35 to 40 minutes, uncovered, until thickened and browned.

5. Cut into 8 squares and serve warm.

Nutrition : Calories: 138; Total Fat: 3g; Saturated Fat: 1g; Protein: 6g; Carbs: 22g; Sugar: 10g; Fiber: 3g; Cholesterol: 24mg; Sodium: 191mg

Steel-Cut Oatmeal Bowl With Fruit And Nuts

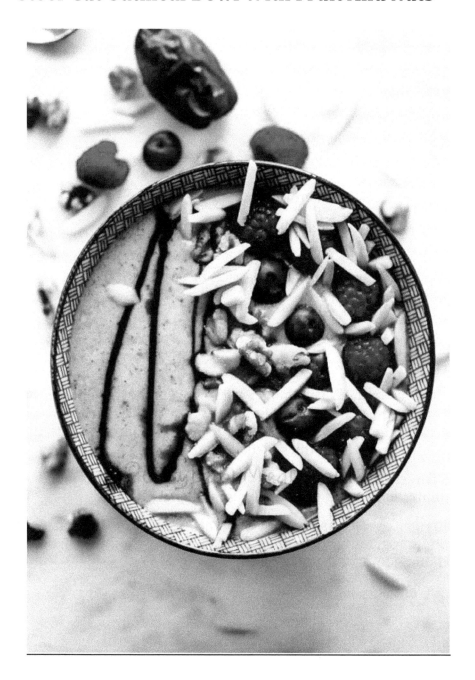

Preparation Time : 5 minutes

Cooking Time : 20 minutes

Servings : 4

Ingredients:

- 1 cup steel-cut oats

- 2 cups almond milk

- ¾ cup water

- 1 teaspoon ground cinnamon

- ¼ teaspoon salt

- 2 cups chopped fresh fruit, such as blueberries, strawberries, raspberries, or peaches

- 1/2 cup chopped walnuts

- ¼ cup chia seeds

Directions :

1. In a medium saucepan over medium-high heat, combine the oats, almond milk, water, cinnamon, and salt. Bring to a boil, reduce the heat to low, and simmer for 15 to 20 minutes, until the oats are softened and thickened.

2. Top each bowl with 1/2 cup of fresh fruit, 2 tablespoons of walnuts, and 1 tablespoon of chia seeds before serving.

Nutrition : Calories: 288; Total Fat: 11g; Saturated Fat: 1g; Protein: 10g; Carbs: 38g; Sugar: 7g; Fiber: 10g; Cholesterol: 0mg; Sodium: 329mg

Whole-Grain Dutch Baby Pancake

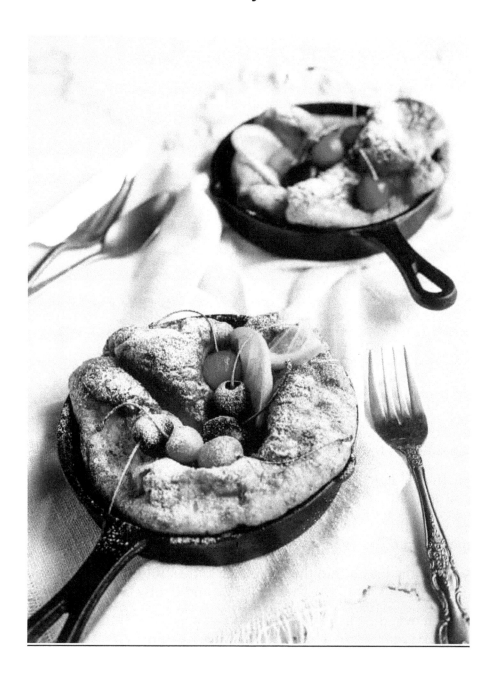

Preparation Time : 5 minutes

Cooking Time : 25 minutes

Servings : 4

Ingredients :

- 2 tablespoons coconut oil
- 1/2 cup whole-wheat flour
- ¼ cup skim milk
- 3 large eggs
- 1 teaspoon vanilla extract
- 1/2 teaspoon baking powder
- ¼ teaspoon salt
- ¼ teaspoon ground cinnamon
- Powdered sugar, for dusting

Directions :

1. Preheat the oven to 400f.

2. Put the coconut oil in a medium oven-safe skillet, and place the skillet in the oven to melt the oil while it preheats.

3. In a blender, combine the flour, milk, eggs, vanilla, baking powder, salt, and cinnamon. Process until smooth.

4. Carefully remove the skillet from the oven and tilt to spread the oil around evenly.

5. Pour the batter into the skillet and return it to the oven for 23 to 25 minutes, until the pancake puffs and lightly browns.

6. Remove, dust lightly with powdered sugar, cut into 4 wedges, and serve.

Nutrition : Calories: 195; Total Fat: 11g; Saturated Fat: 7g; Protein: 8g; Carbs: 16g; Sugar: 1g; Fiber: 2g; Cholesterol: 140mg; Sodium: 209mg

Mushroom, Zucchini, And Onion Frittata

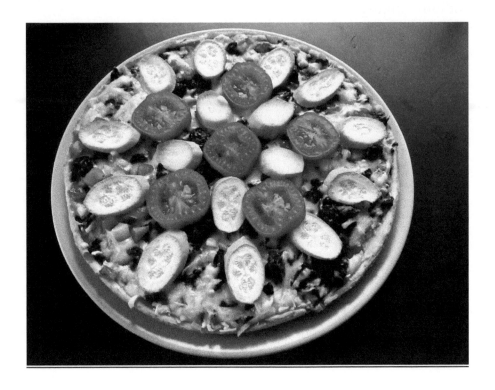

Preparation Time : 10 minutes

Cooking Time : 20 minutes

Servings : 4

Ingredients:

- 1 tablespoon extra-virgin olive oil
- 1/2 onion, chopped
- 1 medium zucchini, chopped
- 11/2 cups sliced mushrooms
- 6 large eggs, beaten
- 2 tablespoons skim milk
- Salt
- Freshly ground black pepper
- 1 ounce feta cheese, crumbled

Directions :

1. Preheat the oven to 400f.

2. In a medium oven-safe skillet over medium-high heat, heat the olive oil.

3. Add the onion and sauté for 3 to 5 minutes, until translucent.

4. Add the zucchini and mushrooms, and cook for 3 to 5 more minutes, until the vegetables are tender.

5. Meanwhile, in a small bowl, whisk the eggs, milk, salt, and pepper. Pour the mixture into the skillet, stirring to combine, and transfer the skillet to the oven. Cook for 7 to 9 minutes, until set.

6. Sprinkle with the feta cheese, and cook for 1 to 2 minutes more, until heated through.

7. Remove, cut into 4 wedges, and serve.

Nutrition : Calories: 178; Total Fat: 13g; Saturated Fat: 4g; Protein: 12g; Carbs: 5g; Sugar: 3g; Fiber: 1g; Cholesterol: 285mg; Sodium: 234mg

Spinach And Cheese Quiche

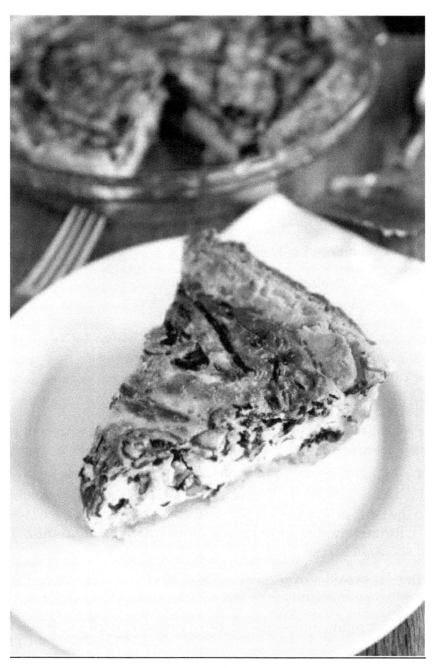

Preparation Time : 10 minutes, plus 10 minutes to rest

Cooking Time : 50 minutes

Servings : 4 to 6

Ingredients:

- Nonstick cooking spray
- 8 ounces yukon gold potatoes, shredded
- 1 tablespoon plus 2 teaspoons extra-virgin olive oil, divided
- 1 teaspoon salt, divided
- Freshly ground black pepper
- 1 onion, finely chopped
- 1 (10-ounce) bag fresh spinach
- 4 large eggs
- 1/2 cup skim milk
- 1 ounce gruyere cheese, shredded

Directions :

1. Preheat the oven to 350f. Spray a 9-inch pie dish with cooking spray. Set aside.

2. In a small bowl, toss the potatoes with 2 teaspoons of olive oil, 1/2 teaspoon of salt, and season with pepper. Press the potatoes into the bottom and sides of the pie dish to form a thin, even layer. Bake for 20 minutes, until golden brown. Remove from the oven and set aside to cool.

3. In a large skillet over medium-high heat, heat the remaining 1 tablespoon of olive oil.

4. Add the onion and sauté for 3 to 5 minutes, until softened.

5. By handfuls, add the spinach, stirring between each addition, until it just starts to wilt before adding more. Cook for about 1 minute, until it cooks down.

6. In a medium bowl, whisk the eggs and milk. Add the gruyere, and season with the remaining 1/2 teaspoon of salt and some pepper. Fold the eggs into the spinach. Pour the mixture into the pie dish and bake for 25 minutes, until the eggs are set.

7. Let rest for 10 minutes before serving.

Nutrition : Calories: 445; Total Fat: 14g; Saturated Fat: 4g; Protein: 19g; Carbs: 68g; Sugar: 6g; Fiber: 7g; Cholesterol: 193mg; Sodium: 773mg

Spicy Jalapeno Popper Deviled Eggs

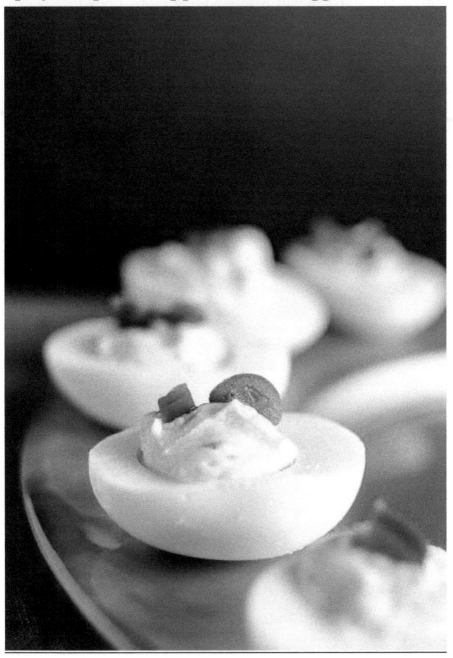

Preparation Time : 5 minutes

Cooking Time : 5 minutes

Servings : 4

Ingredients :

- 4 large whole eggs, hardboiled
- 2 tablespoons Keto-Friendly mayonnaise
- ¼ cup cheddar cheese, grated
- 2 slices bacon, cooked and crumbled
- 1 jalapeno, sliced

Directions :

1. Cut eggs in half, remove the yolk and put them in bowl
2. Lay egg whites on a platter
3. Mix in remaining ingredients and mash them with the egg yolks
4. Transfer yolk mix back to the egg whites
5. Serve and enjoy!

Nutrition : Calories: 176; Fat: 14g; Carbohydrates: 0.7g; Protein: 10g

Lovely Porridge

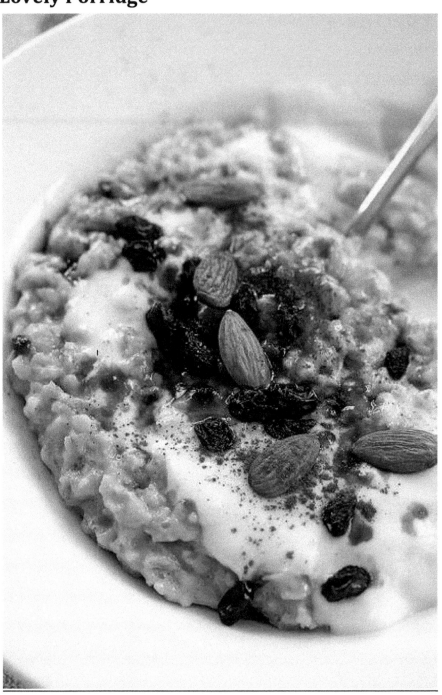

Preparation Time : 15 minutes

Cooking Time : Nil

Servings : 2

Ingredients:

- 2 tablespoons coconut flour
- 2 tablespoons vanilla protein powder
- 3 tablespoons Golden Flaxseed meal
- 1 and 1/2 cups almond milk, unsweetened
- Powdered erythritol

Directions :

1. Take a bowl and mix in flaxseed meal, protein powder, coconut flour and mix well
2. Add mix to the saucepan (placed over medium heat)
3. Add almond milk and stir, let the mixture thicken
4. Add your desired amount of sweetener and serve
5. Enjoy!

Nutrition : Calories: 259; Fat: 13g; Carbohydrates: 5g; Protein: 16g

Salty Macadamia Chocolate Smoothie

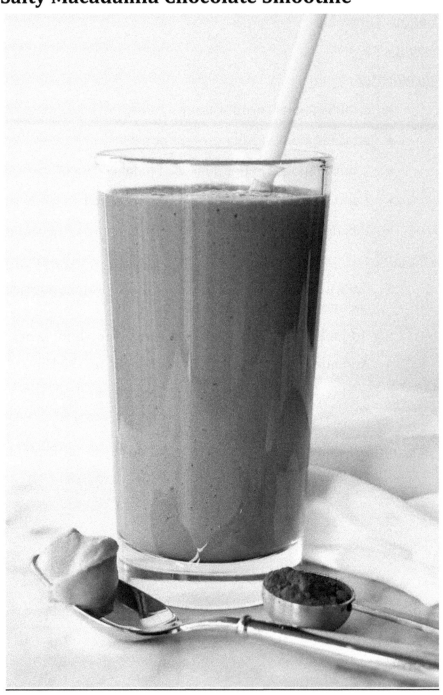

Preparation Time : 5 minutes

Cooking Time : Nil

Servings : 1

Ingredients :

- 2 tablespoons macadamia nuts, salted
- 1/3 cup chocolate whey protein powder, low carb
- 1 cup almond milk, unsweetened

Directions :

1. Add the listed ingredients to your blender and blend until you have a smooth mixture
2. Chill and enjoy it!

Nutrition : Calories: 165; Fat: 2g; Carbohydrates: 1g; Protein: 12g

Basil and Tomato Baked Eggs

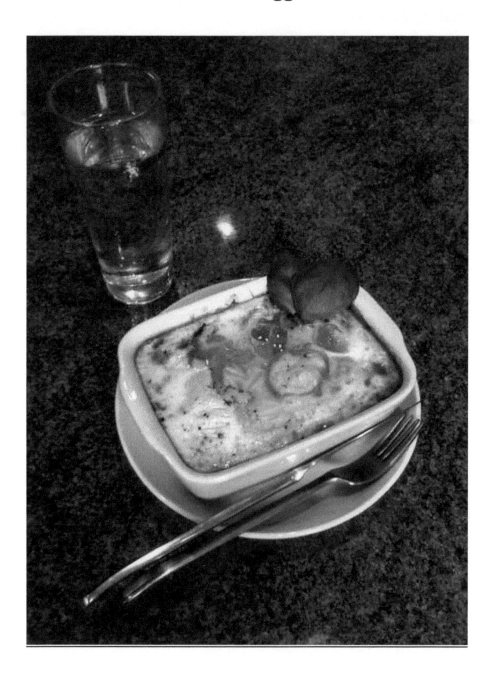

Preparation Time : 10 minutes

Cooking Time : 15 minutes

Servings : 4

Ingredients:

- 1 garlic clove, minced

- 1 cup canned tomatoes

- ¼ cup fresh basil leaves, roughly chopped

- 1/2 teaspoon chili powder

- 1 tablespoon olive oil

- 4 whole eggs

- Salt and pepper to taste

Directions :

1. Preheat your oven to 375 degrees F

2. Take a small baking dish and grease with olive oil

3. Add garlic, basil, tomatoes chili, olive oil into a dish and stir

4. Crackdown eggs into a dish, keeping space between the two

5. Sprinkle the whole dish with salt and pepper

6. Place in oven and cook for 12 minutes until eggs are set and tomatoes are bubbling

7. Serve with basil on top

8. Enjoy!

Nutrition : Calories: 235; Fat: 16g; Carbohydrates: 7g; Protein: 14g

Cinnamon and Coconut Porridge

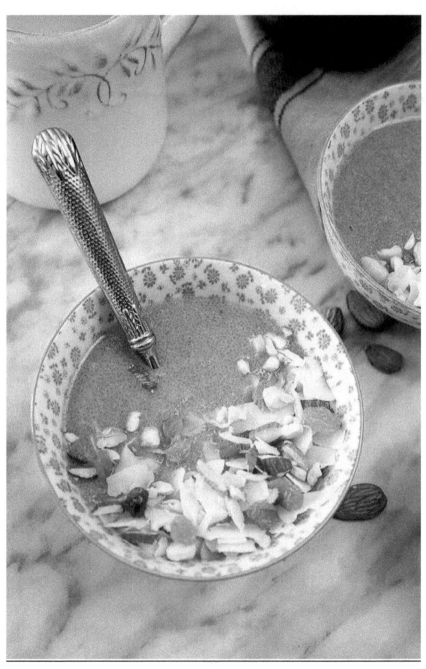

Preparation Time : 5 minutes

Cooking Time : 5 minutes

Servings : 4

Ingredients:

- 2 cups of water
- 1 cup 36% heavy cream
- 1/2 cup unsweetened dried coconut, shredded
- 2 tablespoons flaxseed meal
- 1 tablespoon butter
- 1 and 1/2 teaspoon stevia
- 1 teaspoon cinnamon
- Salt to taste
- Toppings as blueberries

Directions :

1. Add the listed ingredients to a small pot, mix well
2. Transfer pot to stove and place it over medium-low heat
3. Bring to mix to a slow boil
4. Stir well and remove the heat
5. Divide the mix into equal servings and let them sit for 10 minutes
6. Top with your desired toppings and enjoy!

Nutrition : Calories: 171; Fat: 16g; Carbohydrates: 6g; Protein: 2g

An Omelet of Swiss chard

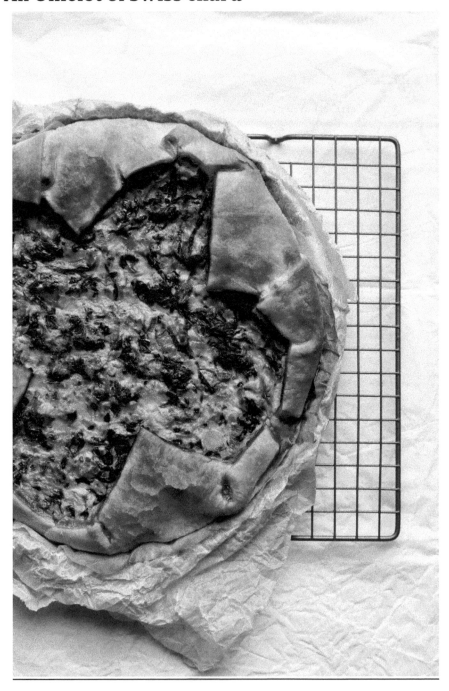

Preparation Time : 5 minutes

Cooking Time : 5 minutes

Servings : 4

Ingredients:

- 4 eggs, lightly beaten
- 4 cups Swiss chard, sliced
- 2 tablespoons butter
- 1/2 teaspoon garlic salt
- Fresh pepper

Directions :

1. Take a non-stick frying pan and place it over medium-low heat
2. Once the butter melts, add Swiss chard and stir cook for 2 minutes
3. Pour egg into the pan and gently stir them into Swiss chard
4. Season with garlic salt and pepper
5. Cook for 2 minutes
6. Serve and enjoy!

Nutrition : Calories: 260; Fat: 21g; Carbohydrates: 4g; Protein: 14g

Cheesy Low-Carb Omelet

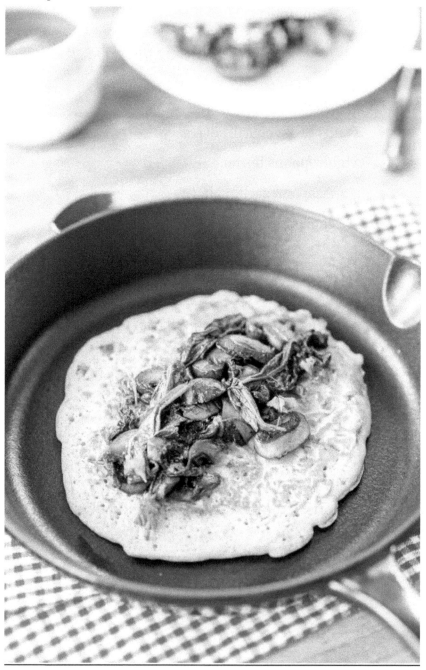

Preparation Time : 5 minutes

Cooking Time : 5 minutes

Servings : 5

Ingredients:

- 2 whole eggs
- 1 tablespoon water
- 1 tablespoon butter
- 3 thin slices salami
- 5 fresh basil leaves
- 5 thin slices, fresh ripe tomatoes
- 2 ounces fresh mozzarella cheese
- Salt and pepper as needed

Directions:

1. Take a small bowl and whisk in eggs and water
2. Take a non-stick Sauté pan and place it over medium heat, add butter and let it melt
3. Pour egg mixture and cook for 30 seconds
4. Spread salami slices on half of egg mix and top with cheese, tomatoes, basil slices
5. Season with salt and pepper according to your taste
6. Cook for 2 minutes and fold the egg with the empty half
7. Cover and cook on LOW for 1 minute
8. Serve and enjoy!

Nutrition : Calories: 451; Fat: 36g; Carbohydrates: 3g; Protein:33g

Yogurt and Kale Smoothie

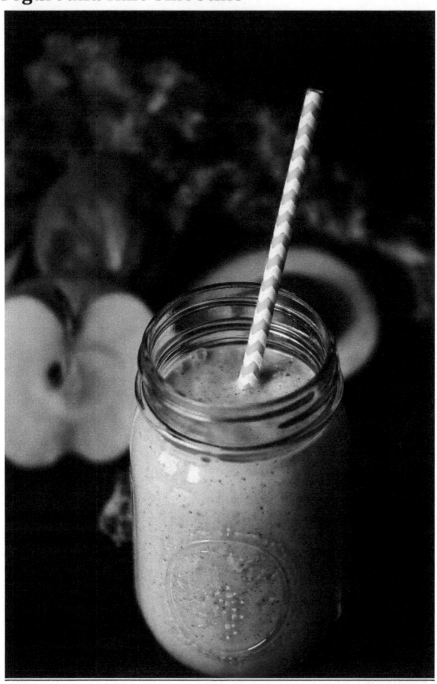

Servings : 1

Preparation Time : 10 minutes

Ingredients:

- 1 cup whole milk yogurt
- 1 cup baby kale greens
- 1 pack stevia
- 1 tablespoon MCT oil
- 1 tablespoon sunflower seeds
- 1 cup of water

Directions :

1. Add listed ingredients to the blender
2. Blend until you have a smooth and creamy texture
3. Serve chilled and enjoy!

Nutrition : Calories: 329; Fat: 26g; Farbohydrates: 15g; Protein: 11g

Bacon and Chicken Garlic Wrap

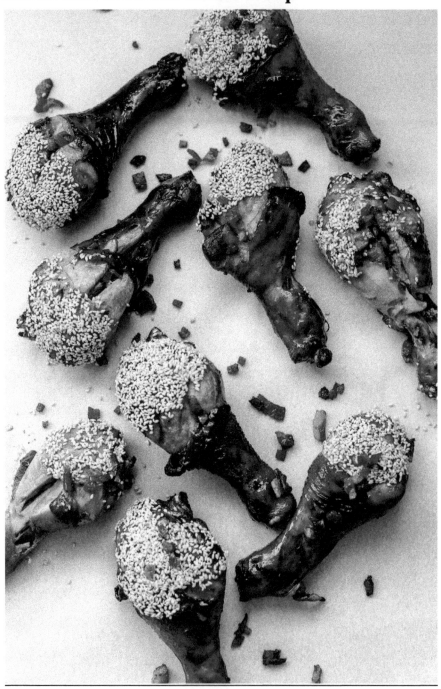

Preparation Time : 15 minutes

Cooking Time : 10 minutes

Servings : 4

Ingredients :

- 1 chicken fillet, cut into small cubes
- 8-9 thin slices bacon, cut to fit cubes
- 6 garlic cloves, minced

Directions :

1. Preheat your oven to 400 degrees F
2. Line a baking tray with aluminum foil
3. Add minced garlic to a bowl and rub each chicken piece with it
4. Wrap bacon piece around each garlic chicken bite
5. Secure with toothpick
6. Transfer bites to the baking sheet, keeping a little bit of space between them
7. Bake for about 15-20 minutes until crispy
8. Serve and enjoy!

Nutrition : Calories: 260; Fat: 19g; Carbohydrates: 5g; Protein: 22g

Grilled Chicken Platter

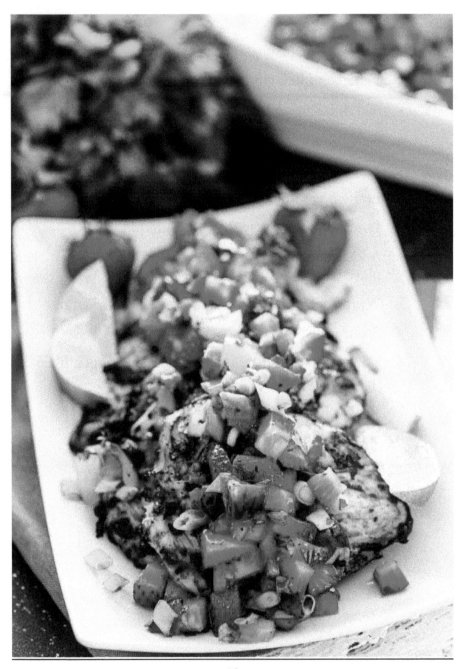

Preparation Time : 5 minutes

Cooking Time : 10 minutes

Servings : 6

Ingredients:

- 3 large chicken breasts, sliced half lengthwise
- 10-ounce spinach, frozen and drained
- 3-ounce mozzarella cheese, part-skim
- 1/2 a cup of roasted red peppers, cut in long strips
- 1 teaspoon of olive oil
- 2 garlic cloves, minced
- Salt and pepper as needed

Directions :

1. Preheat your oven to 400 degrees Fahrenheit
2. Slice 3 chicken breast lengthwise
3. Take a non-stick pan and grease with cooking spray
4. Bake for 2-3 minutes each side
5. Take another skillet and cook spinach and garlic in oil for 3 minutes
6. Place chicken on an oven pan and top with spinach, roasted peppers, and mozzarella
7. Bake until the cheese melted
8. Enjoy!

Nutrition : Calories: 195; Fat: 7g; Net Carbohydrates: 3g; Protein: 30g

Parsley Chicken Breast

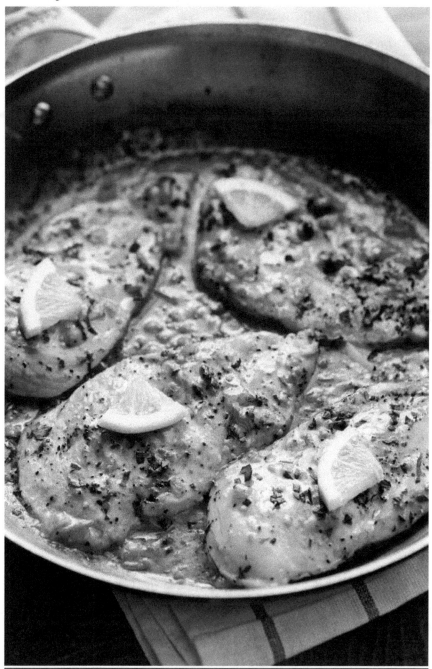

Preparation Time : 10 minutes

Cooking Time : 40 minutes

Servings : 4

Ingredients:

- 1 tablespoon dry parsley
- 1 tablespoon dry basil
- 4 chicken breast halves, boneless and skinless
- 1/2 teaspoon salt
- 1/2 teaspoon red pepper flakes, crushed
- 2 tomatoes, sliced

Directions :

1. Preheat your oven to 350 degrees F
2. Take a 9x13 inch baking dish and grease it up with cooking spray
3. Sprinkle 1 tablespoon of parsley, 1 teaspoon of basil and spread the mixture over your baking dish
4. Arrange the chicken breast halves over the dish and sprinkle garlic slices on top
5. Take a small bowl and add 1 teaspoon parsley, 1 teaspoon of basil, salt, basil, red pepper and mix well. Pour the mixture over the chicken breast
6. Top with tomato slices and cover, bake for 25 minutes
7. Remove the cover and bake for 15 minutes more
8. Serve and enjoy!

Nutrition : Calories: 150; Fat: 4g; Carbohydrates: 4g; Protein: 25g

Mustard Chicken

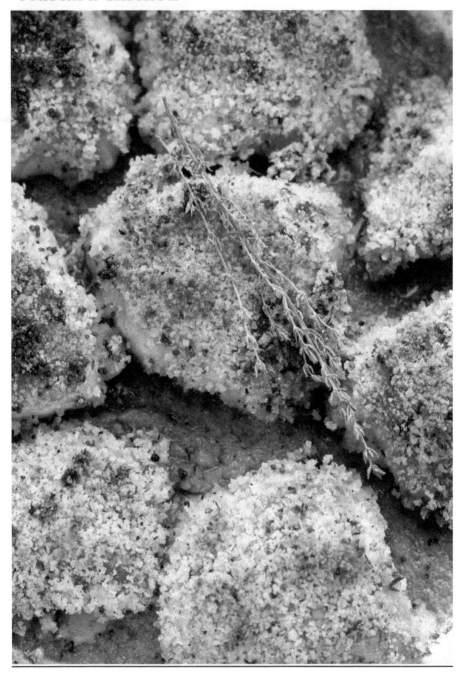

Preparation Time : 10 minutes

Cooking Time : 40 minutes

Servings : 4

Ingredients:

- 4 chicken breasts
- 1/2 cup chicken broth
- 3-4 tablespoons mustard
- 3 tablespoons olive oil
- 1 teaspoon paprika
- 1 teaspoon chili powder
- 1 teaspoon garlic powder

Directions :

1. Take a small bowl and mix mustard, olive oil, paprika, chicken broth, garlic powder, chicken broth, and chili
2. Add chicken breast and marinate for 30 minutes
3. Take a lined baking sheet and arrange the chicken
4. Bake for 35 minutes at 375 degrees Fahrenheit
5. Serve and enjoy!

Nutrition : Calories: 531; Fat: 23g; Carbohydrates: 10g; Protein: 64g

Balsamic Chicken

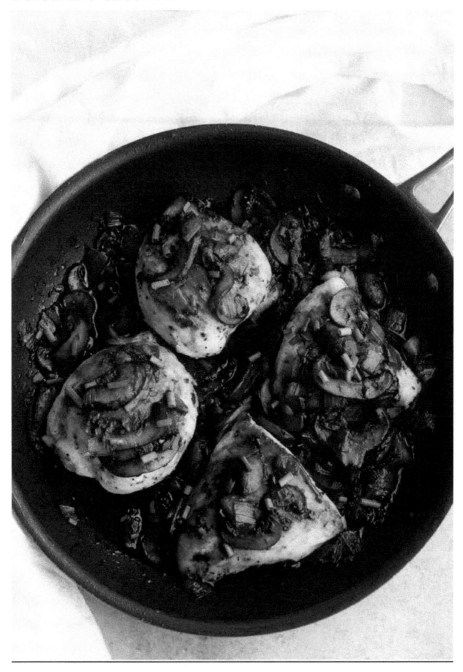

Preparation Time : 10 minutes

Cooking Time : 25 minutes

Servings : 6

Ingredients :

- 6 chicken breast halves, skinless and boneless
- 1 teaspoon garlic salt
- Ground black pepper
- 2 tablespoons olive oil
- 1 onion, thinly sliced
- 14- and 1/2-ounces tomatoes, diced
- 1/2 cup balsamic vinegar
- 1 teaspoon dried basil
- 1 teaspoon dried oregano
- 1 teaspoon dried rosemary
- 1/2 teaspoon dried thyme

Directions :

1. Season both sides of your chicken breasts thoroughly with pepper and garlic salt
2. Take a skillet and place it over medium heat
3. Add some oil and cook your seasoned chicken for 3-4 minutes per side until the breasts are nicely browned
4. Add some onion and cook for another 3-4 minutes until the onions are browned
5. Pour the diced-up tomatoes and balsamic vinegar over your chicken and season with some rosemary, basil, thyme, and rosemary

6. Simmer the chicken for about 15 minutes until they are no longer pink

7. Take an instant-read thermometer and check if the internal temperature gives a reading of 165 degrees Fahrenheit

8. If yes, then you are good to go!

Nutrition : Calories: 196; Fat: 7g; Carbohydrates: 7g; Protein: 23g

Greek Chicken Breast

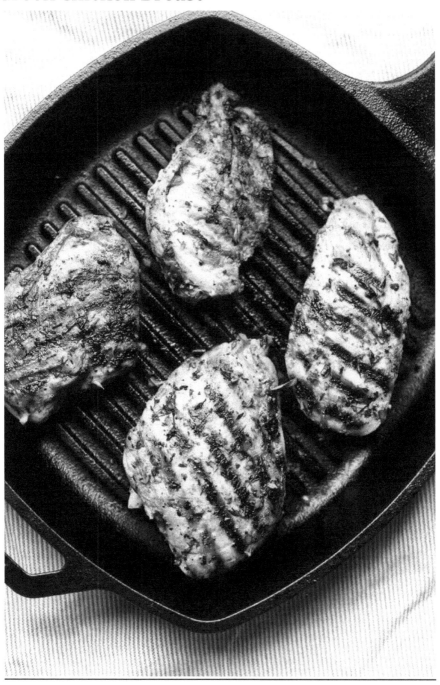

Preparation Time : 10 minutes

Cooking Time : 25 minutes

Servings : 4

Ingredients:

- 4 chicken breast halves, skinless and boneless
- 1 cup extra virgin olive oil
- 1 lemon, juiced
- 2 teaspoons garlic, crushed
- 1 and 1/2 teaspoons black pepper
- 1/3 teaspoon paprika

Directions :

1. Cut 3 slits in the chicken breast
2. Take a small bowl and whisk in olive oil, salt, lemon juice, garlic, paprika, pepper and whisk for 30 seconds
3. Place chicken in a large bowl and pour marinade
4. Rub the marinade all over using your hand
5. Refrigerate overnight
6. Pre-heat grill to medium heat and oil the grate
7. Cook chicken in the grill until center is no longer pink
8. Serve and enjoy!

Nutrition : Calories: 644; Fat: 57g; Carbohydrates: 2g; Protein: 27g

Chipotle Lettuce Chicken

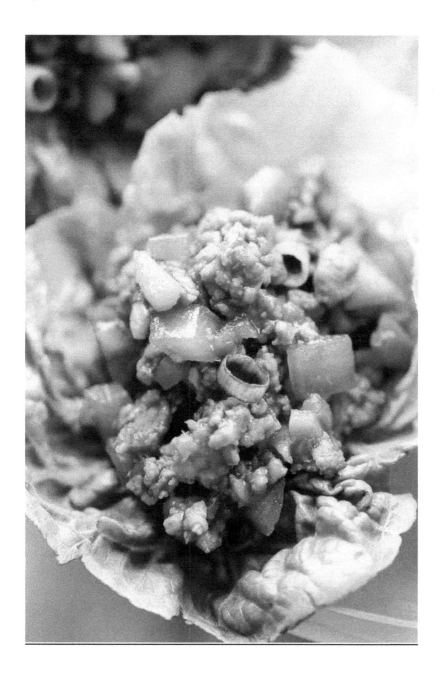

Preparation Time : 10 minutes

Cooking Time : 25 minutes

Servings : 6

Ingredients:

- 1 pound chicken breast, cut into strips
- Splash of olive oil
- 1 red onion, finely sliced
- 14 ounces tomatoes
- 1 teaspoon chipotle, chopped
- 1/2 teaspoon cumin
- Pinch of sugar
- Lettuce as needed
- Fresh coriander leaves
- Jalapeno chilies, sliced
- Fresh tomato slices for garnish
- Lime wedges

Directions :

1. Take a non-stick frying pan and place it over medium heat

2. Add oil and heat it up

3. Add chicken and cook until brown

4. Keep the chicken on the side

5. Add tomatoes, sugar, chipotle, cumin to the same pan and simmer for 25 minutes until you have a nice sauce

6. Add chicken into the sauce and cook for 5 minutes

7. Transfer the mix to another place

8. Use lettuce wraps to take a portion of the mixture and serve with a squeeze of lemon

9. Enjoy!

Nutrition : Calories: 332; Fat: 15g; Carbohydrates: 13g; Protein: 34g

Stylish Chicken-Bacon Wrap

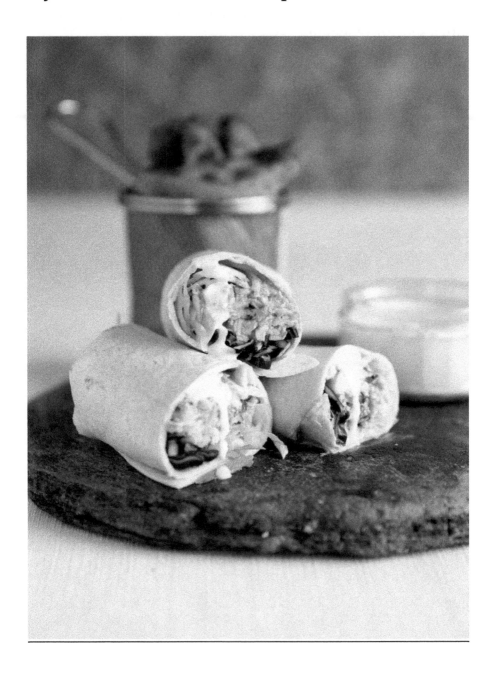

Preparation Time : 5 minutes

Cooking Time : 50 minutes

Servings : 3

Ingredients:

- 8 ounces lean chicken breast
- 6 bacon slices
- 3 ounces shredded cheese
- 4 slices ham

Directions:

1. Cut chicken breast into bite-sized portions
2. Transfer shredded cheese onto ham slices
3. Roll up chicken breast and ham slices in bacon slices
4. Take a skillet and place it over medium heat
5. Add olive oil and brown bacon for a while
6. Remove rolls and transfer to your oven
7. Bake for 45 minutes at 325 degrees F
8. Serve and enjoy!

Nutrition : Calories: 275; Fat: 11g; Carbohydrates: 0.5g; Protein: 40g

Healthy Cottage Cheese Pancakes

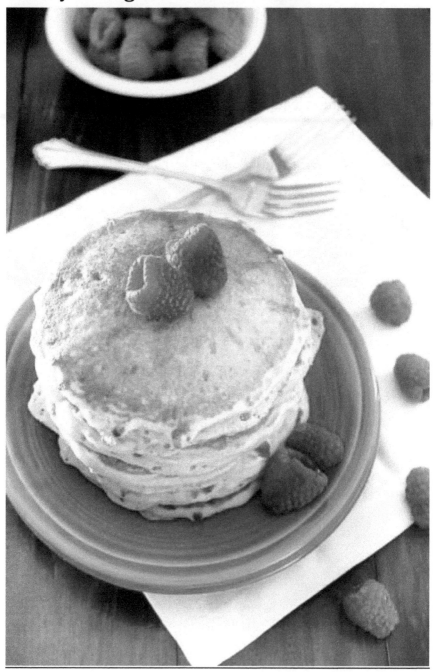

Preparation Time : 10 minutes

Cooking Time : 15

Servings : 1

Ingredients :

- 1/2 cup of Cottage cheese (low-fat)
- 1/3 cup (approx. 2 egg whites) Egg whites
- ¼ cup of Oats
- 1 teaspoon of Vanilla extract
- Olive oil cooking spray
- 1 tablespoon of Stevia (raw)
- Berries or sugar-free jam (optional)

Directions :

1. Begin by taking a food blender and adding in the egg whites and cottage cheese. Also add in the vanilla extract, a pinch of stevia, and oats. Palpitate until the consistency is well smooth.

2. Get a nonstick pan and oil it nicely with the cooking spray. Position the pan on low heat.

3. After it has been heated, scoop out half of the batter and pour it on the pan. Cook for about 21/2 minutes on each side.

4. Position the cooked pancakes on a serving plate and cover with sugar-free jam or berries.

Nutrition : Calories: 205 calories per serving fat – 1.5 g, Protein – 24.5 g, Carbohydrates – 19 g

Avocado Lemon Toast

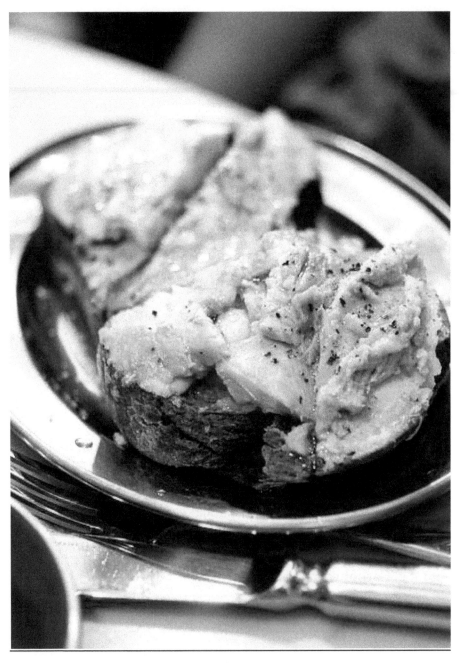

Preparation Time : 10 minutes

Cooking Time : 13 minutes

Servings : 2

Ingredients :

- Whole-grain bread – 2 slices
- Fresh cilantro (chopped) – 2 tablespoons
- Lemon zest – ¼ teaspoon
- Fine sea salt – 1 pinch
- Avocado – 1/2
- Fresh lemon juice – 1 teaspoon
- Cayenne pepper – 1 pinch
- Chia seeds – ¼ teaspoon

Directions :

1. Begin by getting a medium-sized mixing bowl and adding in the avocado. Make use of a fork to crush it properly.

2. Then, add in the cilantro, lemon zest, lemon juice, sea salt, and cayenne pepper. Mix well until combined.

3. Toast the bread slices in a toaster until golden brown. It should take about 3 minutes.

4. Top the toasted bread slices with the avocado mixture and finalize by drizzling with chia seeds.

Nutrition : Calories: 72 calories per serving; Protein – 3.6 g; Fat – 1.2 g; Carbohydrates – 11.6 g

Healthy Baked Eggs

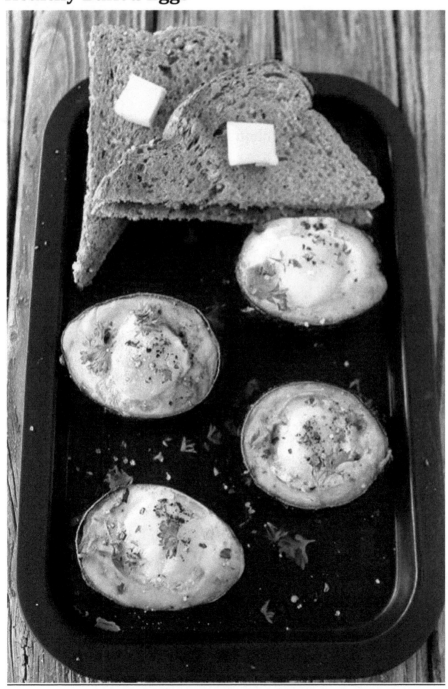

Preparation Time : 10 minutes

Cooking Time : 1 hour

Servings : 6

Ingredients :

- Olive oil – 1 tablespoon
- Garlic – 2 cloves
- Eggs – 8 larges
- Sea salt – 1/2 teaspoon
- Shredded mozzarella cheese (medium-fat) – 3 cups
- Olive oil spray
- Onion (chopped) – 1 medium
- Spinach leaves – 8 ounces
- Half-and-half – 1 cup
- Black pepper – 1 teaspoon
- Feta cheese – 1/2 cup

Directions :

1. Begin by heating the oven to 375F.
2. Get a glass baking dish and grease it with olive oil spray. Arrange aside.
3. Now take a nonstick pan and pour in the olive oil. Position the pan on allows heat and allows it heat.
4. Immediately you are done, toss in the garlic, spinach, and onion. Prepare for about 5 minutes. Arrange aside.

5. You can now Get a large mixing bowl and add in the half, eggs, pepper, and salt. Whisk thoroughly to combine.

6. Put in the feta cheese and chopped mozzarella cheese (reserve 1/2 cup of mozzarella cheese for later).

7. Put the egg mixture and prepared spinach to the prepared glass baking dish. Blend well to combine. Drizzle the reserved cheese over the top.

8. Bake the egg mix for about 45 minutes.

9. Extract the baking dish from the oven and allow it to stand for 10 minutes.

10. Dice and serve!

Nutrition : Calories: 323 calories per serving;Fat – 22.3 g; Protein – 22.6 g; Carbohydrates – 7.9 g

Quick Low-Carb Oatmeal

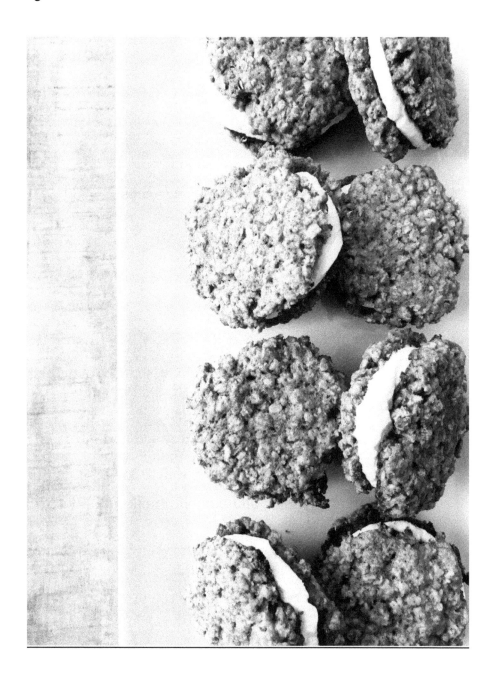

Preparation Time : 10 minutes

Cooking Time : 15 minutes

Servings : 2

Ingredients :

- Almond flour – 1/2 cup
- Flax meal – 2 tablespoons
- Cinnamon (ground) – 1 teaspoon
- Almond milk (unsweetened) – 11/2 cups
- Salt – as per taste
- Chia seeds – 2 tablespoons
- Liquid stevia – 10 – 15 drops
- Vanilla extract – 1 teaspoon

Directions :

1. Begin by taking a large mixing bowl and adding in the coconut flour, almond flour, ground cinnamon, flax seed powder, and chia seeds. Mix properly to combine.

2. Position a stockpot on a low heat and add in the dry ingredients. Also add in the liquid stevia, vanilla extract, and almond milk. Mix well to combine.

3. Prepare the flour and almond milk for about 4 minutes. Add salt if needed.

4. Move the oatmeal to a serving bowl and top with nuts, seeds, and pure and neat berries.

Nutrition : Calories: calories per serving; Protein – 11.7 g; Fat – 24.3 g; Carbohydrates – 16.7 g

Tofu and Vegetable Scramble

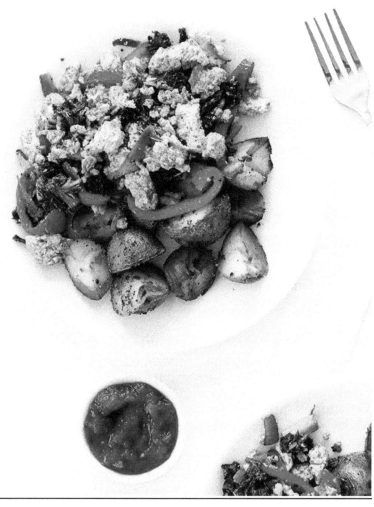

Preparation Time : 10 minutes

Cooking Time : 15 minutes

Servings : 2

Ingredients :

- Firm tofu (drained) – 16 ounces
- Sea salt – 1/2 teaspoon
- Garlic powder – 1 teaspoon
- Fresh coriander – for garnishing
- Red onion – 1/2 medium
- Cumin powder – 1 teaspoon
- Lemon juice – for topping
- Green bell pepper – 1 medium
- Garlic powder – 1 teaspoon
- Fresh coriander – for garnishing
- Red onion – 1/2 medium
- Cumin powder – 1 teaspoon
- Lemon juice – for topping

Directions :

1. Begin by preparing the ingredients. For this, you are to extract the seeds of the tomato and green bell pepper. Shred the onion, bell pepper, and tomato into small cubes.

2. Get a small mixing bowl and position the fairly hard tofu inside it. Make use of your hands to break the fairly hard tofu. Arrange aside.

3. Get a nonstick pan and add in the onion, tomato, and bell pepper. Mix and cook for about 3 minutes.

4. Put the somewhat hard crumbled tofu to the pan and combine well.

5. Get a small bowl and put in the water, turmeric, garlic powder, cumin powder, and chili powder. Combine well and stream it over the tofu and vegetable mixture.

6. Allow the tofu and vegetable crumble cook with seasoning for 5 minutes. Continuously stir so that the pan is not holding the ingredients.

7. Drizzle the tofu scramble with chili flakes and salt. Combine well.

8. Transfer the prepared scramble to a serving bowl and give it a proper spray of lemon juice.

9. Finalize by garnishing with pure and neat coriander. Serve while hot!

Nutrition : Calories: 238 calories per serving; Carbohydrates − 16.6 g; Fat − 11 g

Breakfast Smoothie Bowl with Fresh Berries

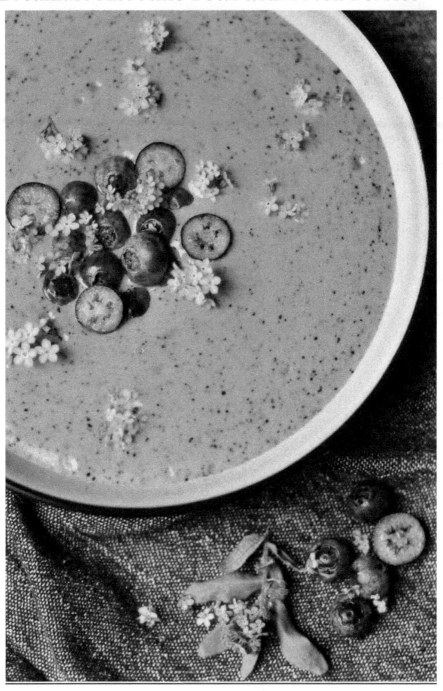

Preparation Time : 10 minutes

Cooking Time : 5 minutes

Servings : 2

Ingredients :

- Almond milk (unsweetened) – 1/2 cup
- Psyllium husk powder – 1/2 teaspoon
- Strawberries (chopped) – 2 ounces
- Coconut oil – 1 tablespoon
- Crushed ice – 3 cups
- Liquid stevia – 5 to 10 drops
- Pea protein powder – 1/3 cup

Directions :

1. Begin by taking a blender and adding in the mashed ice cubes. Allow them to rest for about 30 seconds.

2. Then put in the almond milk, shredded strawberries, pea protein powder, psyllium husk powder, coconut oil, and liquid stevia. Blend well until it turns into a smooth and creamy puree.

3. Vacant the prepared smoothie into 2 glasses.

4. Cover with coconut flakes and pure and neat strawberries.

Nutrition : Calories: 166 calories per serving; Fat – 9.2 g; Carbohydrates – 4.1 g; Protein – 17.6 g

Chia and Coconut Pudding

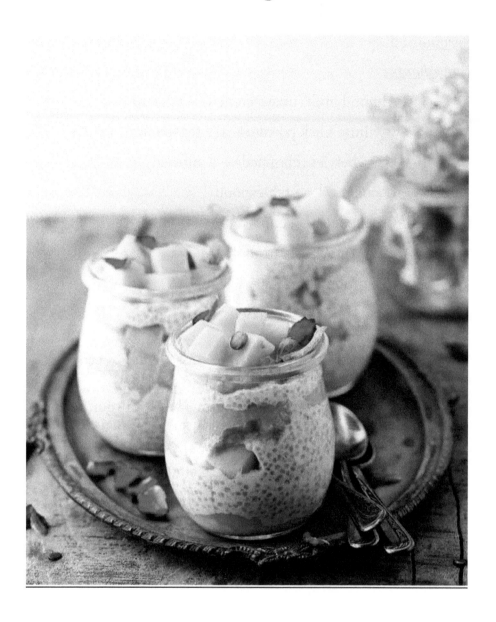

Preparation Time : 10 minutes

Cooking Time : 5 minutes

Servings : 2

Ingredients :

- Light coconut milk – 7 ounces
- Liquid stevia – 3 to 4 drops
- Kiwi – 1
- Chia seeds – ¼ cup
- Clementine – 1
- Shredded coconut (unsweetened)

Directions :

1. Begin by getting a mixing bowl and putting in the light coconut milk. Set in the liquid stevia to sweeten the milk. Combine well.

2. Put the chia seeds to the milk and whisk until well-combined. Arrange aside.

3. Scrape the clementine and carefully extract the skin from the wedges. Leave aside.

4. Also, scrape the kiwi and dice it into small pieces.

5. Get a glass vessel and gather the pudding. For this, position the fruits at the bottom of the jar; then put a dollop of chia pudding. Then spray the fruits and then put another layer of chia pudding.

6. Finalize by garnishing with the rest of the fruits and chopped coconut.

Nutrition : Calories: 201 calories per serving;Protein – 5.4 g; Fat – 10 g; Carbohydrates – 22.8 g

Tomato and Zucchini Sauté

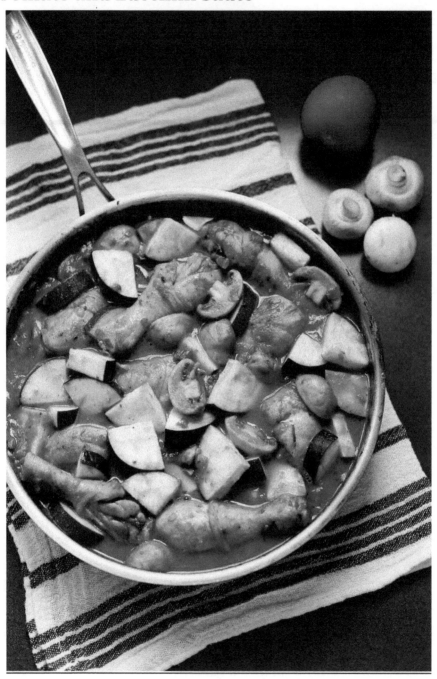

Preparation Time : 10 minutes

Cooking Time : 43 minutes

Servings : 6

Ingredients :

- Vegetable oil – 1 tablespoon

- Tomatoes (chopped) – 2

- Green bell pepper (chopped) – 1

- Black pepper (freshly ground) – as per taste

- Onion (sliced) – 1

- Zucchini (peeled) – 2 pounds and cut into 1-inch-thick slices

- Salt – as per taste

- Uncooked white rice – ¼ cup

Directions :

1. Begin by getting a nonstick pan and putting it over low heat. Stream in the oil and allow it to heat through.

2. Put in the onions and sauté for about 3 minutes.

3. Then pour in the zucchini and green peppers. Mix well and spice with black pepper and salt.

4. Reduce the heat and cover the pan with a lid. Allow the veggies cook on low for 5 minutes.

5. While you're done, put in the water and rice. Place the lid back on and cook on low for 20 minutes.

Nutrition : Calories: 94 calories per serving; Fat – 2.8 g; Protein – 3.2 g; Carbohydrates – 16.1 g

Steamed Kale with Mediterranean Dressing

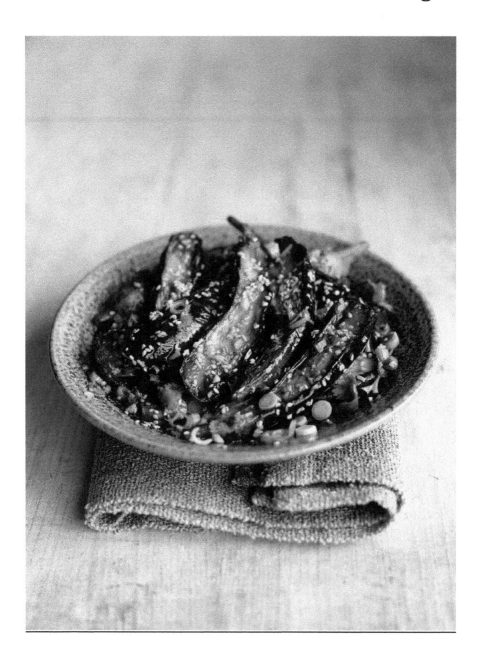

Preparation Time : 10 minutes

Cooking Time : 25 minutes

Servings : 6

Ingredients :

- Kale (chopped) – 12 cups
- Olive oil – 1 tablespoon
- Soy sauce – 1 teaspoon
- Pepper (freshly ground) – as per taste
- Lemon juice – 2 tablespoons
- Garlic (minced) – 1 tablespoon
- Salt – as per taste

Directions :

1. Get a gas steamer or an electric steamer and fill the bottom pan with water. If making use of a gas steamer, position it on high heat. Making use of an electric steamer, place it on the highest setting.

2. Immediately the water comes to a boil, put in the shredded kale and cover with a lid. Boil for about 8 minutes. The kale should be tender by now.

3. During the kale is boiling, take a big mixing bowl and put in the olive oil, lemon juice, soy sauce, garlic, pepper, and salt. Whisk well to mix.

4. Now toss in the steamed kale and carefully enclose into the dressing. Be assured the kale is well-coated.

5. Serve while it's hot!

Nutrition : Calories: 91 calories per serving; Fat – 3.5 g; Protein – 4.6 g; Carbohydrates – 14.5 g

Healthy Carrot Muffins

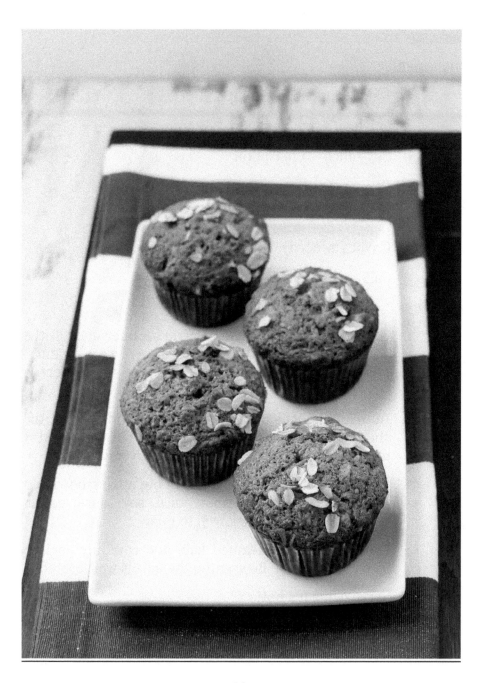

Preparation Time : 10 minutes

Cooking Time : 40 minutes

Servings : 8

Ingredients:

Dry ingredients

- Tapioca starch – ¼ cup
- Baking soda – 1 teaspoon
- Cinnamon – 1 tablespoon
- Cloves – ¼ teaspoon
- Wet ingredients
- Vanilla extract – 1 teaspoon
- Water – 11/2 cups
- Carrots (shredded) – 11/2 cups
- Almond flour – 1¾ cups
- Granulated sweetener of choice – 1/2 cup
- Baking powder – 1 teaspoon
- Nutmeg – 1 teaspoon
- Salt – 1 teaspoon
- Coconut oil – 1/3 cup
- Flax meal – 4 tablespoons
- Banana (mashed) – 1 medium

Directions :

1. Begin by heating the oven to 350F.

2. Get a muffin tray and position paper cups in all the molds. Arrange aside.

3. Get a small glass bowl and put half a cup of water and flax meal. Allow this rest for about 5 minutes. Your flax egg is prepared.

4. Get a large mixing bowl and put in the almond flour, tapioca starch, granulated sugar, baking soda, baking powder, cinnamon, nutmeg, cloves, and salt. Mix well to combine.

5. Conform a well in the middle of the flour mixture and stream in the coconut oil, vanilla extract, and flax egg. Mix well to conform a mushy dough.

Then put in the chopped carrots and mashed banana. Mix until well-combined.

6. Make use of a spoon to scoop out an equal amount of mixture into 8 muffin cups.

7. Position the muffin tray in the oven and allow it to bake for about 40 minutes.

8. Extract the tray from the microwave and allow the muffins to stand for about 10 minutes.

9. Extract the muffin cups from the tray and allow them to chill until they reach room degree of hotness and coldness.

10. Serve and enjoy!

Nutrition : Calories: 189 calories per serving; Fat – 13.9 g; Protein – 3.8 g; Carbohydrates – 17.3 g

Vegetable Noodles Stir-Fry

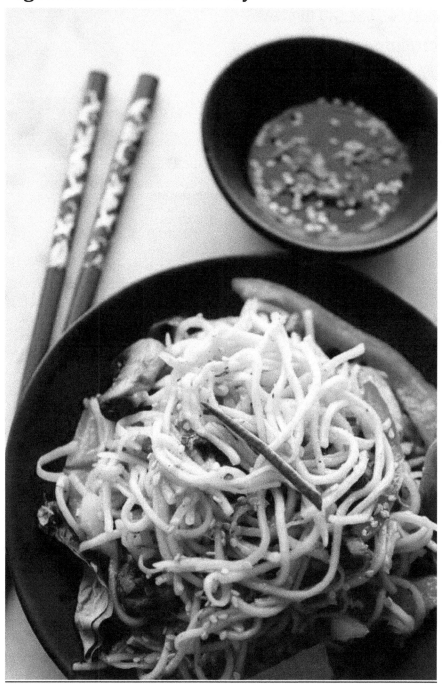

Preparation Time : 10 minutes

Cooking Time : 40 minutes

Servings : 4

Ingredients :

- White sweet potato – 1 pound
- Zucchini – 8 ounces
- Garlic cloves (finely chopped) – 2 large
- Vegetable broth – 2 tablespoons
- Salt – as per taste
- Carrots – 8 ounces
- Shallot (finely chopped) – 1
- Red chili (finely chopped) – 1
- Olive oil – 1 tablespoon
- Pepper – as per taste

Directions :

1. Begin by scrapping the carrots and sweet potato. Make Use a spiralizer to make noodles out of the sweet potato and carrots.

2. Rinse the zucchini thoroughly and spiralize it as well.

3. Get a large skillet and position it on a high flame. Stream in the vegetable broth and allow it to come to a boil.

4. Toss in the spiralized sweet potato and carrots. Then put in the chili, garlic, and shallots. Stir everything using tongs and cook for some minutes.

5. Transfer the vegetable noodles into a serving platter and generously spice with pepper and salt.

6. Finalize by sprinkling olive oil over the noodles. Serve while hot!

Nutrition : Calories: 169 calories per serving; Fat – 3.7 g; Protein – 3.6 g; Carbohydrates – 31.2 g

Cauliflower Mac & Cheese

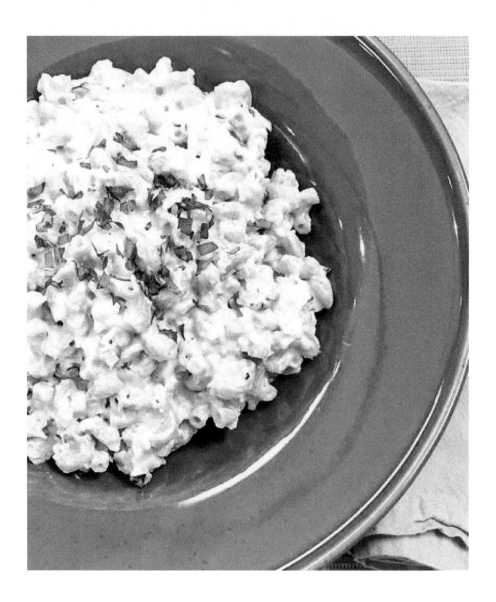

Preparation Time : 5 Minutes

Cooking Time : 25 Minutes

Effort : Easy

Serving Size : 4

Ingredients :

- 1 Cauliflower Head, torn into florets
- Salt & Black Pepper, as needed
- ¼ cup Almond Milk, unsweetened
- ¼ cup Heavy Cream
- 3 tbsp. Butter, preferably grass-fed
- 1 cup Cheddar Cheese, shredded

Directions :

1. Preheat the oven to 450 F.

2. Melt the butter in a small microwave-safe bowl and heat it for 30 seconds.

3. Pour the melted butter over the cauliflower florets along with salt and pepper. Toss them well.

4. Place the cauliflower florets in a parchment paper-covered large baking sheet.

5. Bake them for 15 minutes or until the cauliflower is crisp-tender.

6. Once baked, mix the heavy cream, cheddar cheese, almond milk, and the remaining butter in a large microwave-safe bowl and heat it on high heat for 2 minutes or until the cheese mixture is smooth. Repeat the procedure until the cheese has melted.

7. Finally, stir in the cauliflower to the sauce mixture and coat well.

Nutrition : Calories: 294 kcal; Fat: 23g; Carbohydrates: 7g; Proteins: 11g

Easy Egg Salad

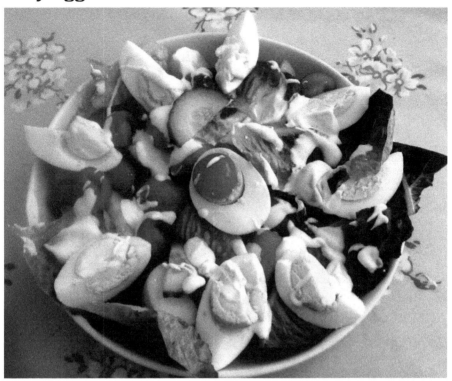

Preparation Time : 5 Minutes

Cooking Time : 15 to 20 Minutes

Effort : Easy

Servings : 4

Ingredients :

- 6 Eggs, preferably free-range
- ¼ tsp. Salt
- 2 tbsp. Mayonnaise
- 1 tsp. Lemon juice
- 1 tsp. Dijon mustard
- Pepper, to taste
- Lettuce leaves, to serve

Directions :

1. Keep the eggs in a saucepan of water and pour cold water until it covers the egg by another 1 inch.
2. Bring to a boil and then remove the eggs from heat.
3. Peel the eggs under cold running water.
4. Transfer the cooked eggs into a food processor and pulse them until chopped.
5. Stir in the mayonnaise, lemon juice, salt, Dijon mustard, and pepper and mix them well.
6. Taste for seasoning and add more if required.
7. Serve in the lettuce leaves.

Nutrition : Calories – 166kcal; Fat – 14g; Carbohydrates - 0.85g; Proteins – 10g; Sodium: 132mg

Baked Chicken Legs

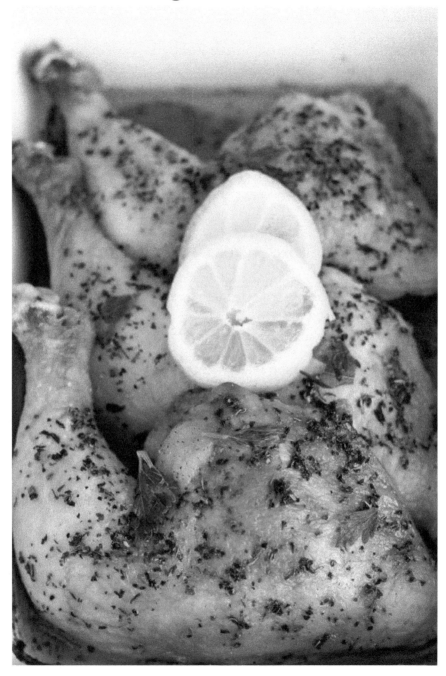

Preparation Time : 10 Minutes

Cooking Time : 40 Minutes

Effort : Easy

Servings : 6

Ingredients :

- 6 Chicken Legs
- ¼ tsp. Black Pepper
- ¼ cup Butter
- 1/2 tsp. Sea Salt
- 1/2 tsp. Smoked Paprika
- 1/2 tsp. Garlic Powder

Directions :

1. Preheat the oven to 425 F.
2. Pat the chicken legs with a paper towel to absorb any excess moisture.
3. Marinate the chicken pieces by first applying the butter over them and then with the seasoning. Set it aside for a few minutes.
4. Bake them for 25 minutes. Turnover and bake for further 10 minutes or until the internal temperature reaches 165 F.
5. Serve them hot.

Nutrition : Calories – 236Kl; Fat – 16g; Carbohydrates – 0g; Protein – 22g;Sodium – 314mg

Creamed Spinach

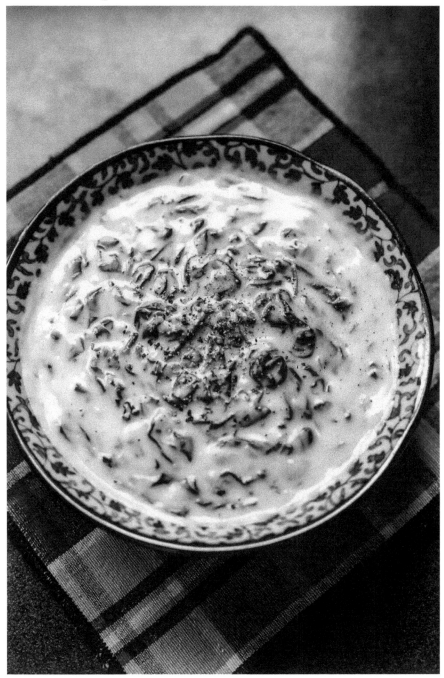

Preparation Time : 5 Minutes

Cooking Time : 10 Minutes

Effort : Easy

Servings : 4

Ingredients :

- 3 tbsp. Butter
- ¼ tsp. Black Pepper
- 4 cloves of Garlic, minced
- ¼ tsp. Sea Salt
- 10 oz. Baby Spinach, chopped
- 1 tsp. Italian Seasoning
- 1/2 cup Heavy Cream
- 3 oz. Cream Cheese

Directions :

1. Melt butter in a large sauté pan over medium heat.

2. Once the butter has melted, spoon in the garlic and sauté for 30 seconds or until aromatic.

3. Spoon in the spinach and cook for 3 to 4 minutes or until wilted.

4. Add all the remaining ingredients to it and continuously stir until the cream cheese melts and the mixture gets thickened.

5. Serve hot

Nutrition : Calories – 274kL; Fat – 27g; Carbohydrates – 4g; Protein – 4g; Sodium – 114mg

Stuffed Mushrooms

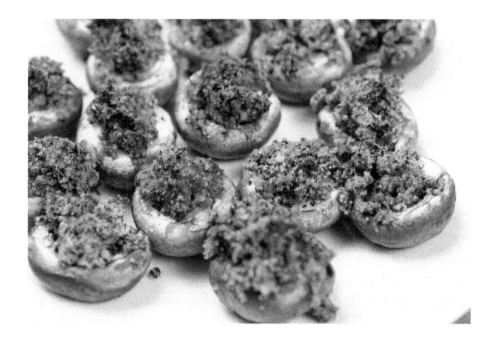

Preparation Time : 10 Minutes

Cooking Time : 20 Minutes

Servings : 4

Ingredients :

- 4 Portobello Mushrooms, large
- 1/2 cup Mozzarella Cheese, shredded
- 1/2 cup Marinara, low-sugar
- Olive Oil Spray

Directions :

1. Preheat the oven to 375 F.
2. Take out the dark gills from the mushrooms with the help of a spoon.
3. Keep the mushroom stem upside down and spoon it with two tablespoons of marinara sauce and mozzarella cheese.
4. Bake for 18 minutes or until the cheese is bubbly.

Nutrition : Calories – 113kL; Fat – 6g; Carbohydrates – 4g; Protein – 7g; Sodium – 14mg

Berry-Oat Breakfast Bars

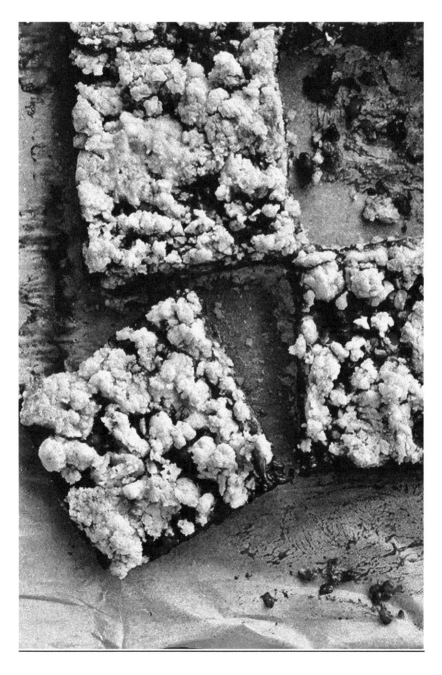

Preparation Time : 10 minutes

Cooking Time : 25 minutes

Servings : 12

Ingredients :

- 2 cups fresh raspberries or blueberries
- 2 tablespoons sugar
- 2 tablespoons freshly squeezed lemon juice
- 1 tablespoon cornstarch
- 11/2 cups rolled oats
- 1/2 cup whole-wheat flour
- 1/2 cup walnuts
- ¼ cup chia seeds
- ¼ cup extra-virgin olive oil
- ¼ cup honey
- 1 large egg

Directions :

1. Preheat the oven to 350f.

2. In a small saucepan over medium heat, stir together the berries, sugar, lemon juice, and cornstarch. Bring to a simmer. Reduce the heat and simmer for 2 to 3 minutes, until the mixture thickens.

3. In a food processor or high-speed blender, combine the oats, flour, walnuts, and chia seeds. Process until powdered. Add the olive oil, honey, and egg. Pulse a few more times, until well combined. Press half of the mixture into a 9-inch square baking dish.

4.   Spread the berry filling over the oat mixture. Add the remaining oat mixture on top of the berries. Bake for 25 minutes, until browned.

5.   Let cool completely, cut into 12 pieces, and serve. Store in a covered container for up to 5 days.

Nutrition : calories: 201; total fat: 10g; saturated fat: 1g; protein: 5g; carbs: 26g; sugar: 9g; fiber: 5g; cholesterol: 16mg; sodium: 8mg

30 minutes or less • nut free • vegetarian

Whole-Grain Breakfast Cookies

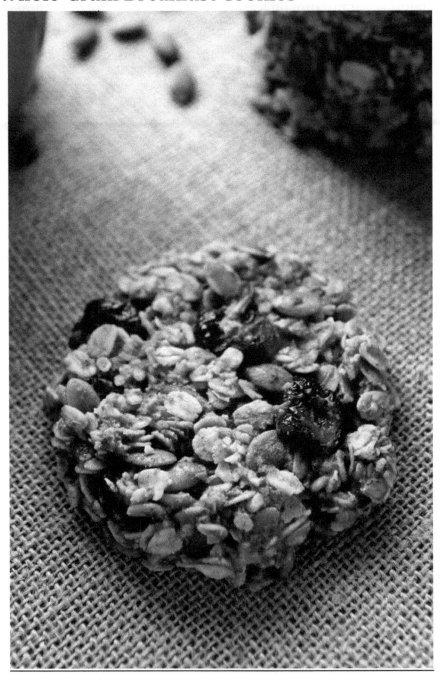

Preparation Time : 20 minutes

Cooking Time : 10 minutes

Servings : 18 cookies

Ingredients :

- 2 cups rolled oats
- 1/2 cup whole-wheat flour
- ¼ cup ground flaxseed
- 1 teaspoon baking powder
- 1 cup unsweetened applesauce
- 2 large eggs
- 2 tablespoons vegetable oil
- 2 teaspoons vanilla extract
- 1 teaspoon ground cinnamon
- 1/2 cup dried cherries
- ¼ cup unsweetened shredded coconut
- 2 ounces dark chocolate, chopped

Directions :

1. Preheat the oven to 350f.

2. In a large bowl, combine the oats, flour, flaxseed, and baking powder. Stir well to mix.

3. In a medium bowl, whisk the applesauce, eggs, vegetable oil, vanilla, and cinnamon. Pour the wet mixture into the dry mixture, and stir until just combined.

4. Fold in the cherries, coconut, and chocolate. Drop tablespoon-size balls of dough onto a baking sheet. Bake for 10 to 12 minutes, until browned and cooked through.

5. Let cool for about 3 minutes, remove from the baking sheet, and cool completely before serving. Store in an airtight container for up to 1 week.

Nutrition : calories: 136; total fat: 7g; saturated fat: 3g; protein: 4g; carbs: 14g; sugar: 4g; fiber: 3g; cholesterol: 21mg; sodium: 11mg

Peanut Butter Bars

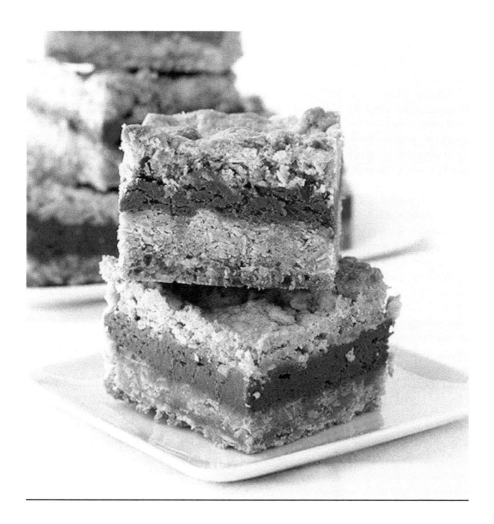

Preparation Time : 10 minutes

Cooking Time : 10 minutes

Servings : 6

Ingredients :

- 3/4 cup almond flour
- 2 oz. almond butter
- 1/4 cup Swerve
- 1/2 cup peanut butter
- 1/2 teaspoon vanilla

Directions :

1. Combine all the Ingredients for bars.
2. Transfer this mixture to 6-inch small pan. Press it firmly.
3. Refrigerate for 30 minutes.
4. Slice and serve.

Nutrition : Calories 214; Total Fat 19 g; Saturated Fat 5.8 g; Cholesterol 15 mg; Total Carbs 6.5 g; Sugar 1.9 g; Fiber 2.1 g; Sodium 123 mg; Protein 6.5 g

Zucchini Bread Pancakes

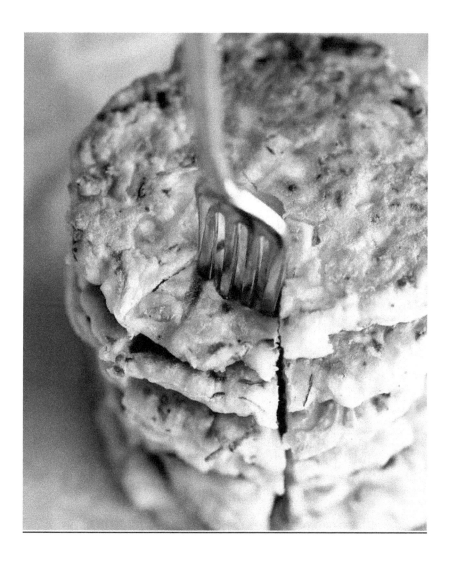

Preparation Time : 15 minutes

Cooking Time : 35 minutes

Servings : 3

Ingredients :

- Grapeseed oil, 1 tbsp.

- Chopped walnuts, .5 c

- Walnut milk, 2 c

- Shredded zucchini, 1 c

- Mashed burro banana, .25 c

- Date sugar, 2 tbsp.

- Kamut flour or spelt, 2 c

Directions :

1. Place the date sugar and flour into a bowl. Whisk together.

2. Add in the mashed banana and walnut milk. Stir until combined. Remember to scrape the bowl to get all the dry mixture. Add in walnuts and zucchini. Stir well until combined.

3. Place the grapeseed oil onto a griddle and warm.

4. Pour .25 cup batter on the hot griddle. Leave it along until bubbles begin forming on to surface. Carefully turn over the pancake and cook another four minutes until cooked through.

5. Place the pancakes onto a serving plate and enjoy with some agave syrup.

Nutrition : Calories: 246; Carbohydrates: 49.2 g; Fiber: 4.6 g; Protein: 7.8

Lightning Source UK Ltd.
Milton Keynes UK
UKHW020637140621
385477UK00005B/69